Revolutionize Your Willpower

The Art of Unbreakable Commitment

Albert Victor Harper

Table of Contents

The difference between a successful person and others is not a lack of strength, not a lack of knowledge, but rather a lack in will.

— Vince Lombardi

Chapter 1. Introduction

Empower your life today with our Special Report: "Revolutionize Your Willpower: The Art of Unbreakable Commitment". Unlock the secrets to transforming your mindset, creating unshakeable resolution, and forging a future that aligns your deepest passions with your day-to-day actions. Steeped in vibrant, enlightening, and practical advice, this illuminating journey dives into the heart of willpower, granting you access to the tools you need to conquer procrastination, overcome doubt, and turn your dreams into reality. This is not just a report; it's your roadmap to personal growth and indomitable perseverance. Discover a life brimming with potential that's merely waiting for your unshakeable commitment. Bursting with enthusiasm? Excellent! Enjoy the sheer bliss of stepping into a new, empowered version of yourself. Asset awaits. Act now to secure this life-changing companion on your path to exceptional willpower. So, are you ready to revolutionize your willpower?

Chapter 2. Understanding the Power of Willpower

The journey starts with the exploration of the essence of willpower. Understanding the power of willpower is akin to acknowledging the bright blazing sun that controls the spin of the planets revolving around it. It's a pivotal internal force that steers our actions and shapes our behaviors, impacting every sphere of life – whether personal or professional.

2.1. Defining Willpower

To appreciate the power of willpower, we first need to grasp its definition. Willpower is essentially the ability to exert self-control, to resist desires, to persevere through the challenges, and to stay committed to achieving long-term goals, despite the odds. It is about making thoughtful choices, caring for the long-term, and avoiding impulsive decisions.

2.2. The Depth, Reach and Influence of Willpower

Willpower is not confined to a single domain. Its reach is broad and it contributes to different aspects of life. A few examples will offer a glimpse into its depth and influence. An individual with robust willpower can resist unhealthy food practices, thus maintaining physical wellbeing. Another person, by stark contrast, may utilize this strength to remain committed to professional growth, working additional hours, or undertaking further education. The common thread here is the ability to postpone immediate gratification for the potential of improved outcomes in the long run. This enduring ability to act in your longer-term interest, instead of immediate desires, is willpower at work. It's a silent power within, steering your decisions and actions often without your conscious recognition, but with enormous consequence.

2.3. Willpower: The Inner Strength

To understand willpower is to recognize it as an inner strength. This strength is not fixed but, rather, can be trained and improved like a muscle. Contrary to popular belief, willpower does not spring from a ferocious, ascetic denial of enjoyment or brute force suppression of desires. It's actually a balanced mix of grit, determination, and the skill to navigate between immediate desires and long-term goals. It is focusing one's energy towards productive and healthy actions, paving the path to success in different areas of life.

2.4. Differentiating Willpower and Motivation

Although seemingly alike, willpower and motivation are two different elements. Motivation is your desire to do something, the "why" behind your actions. It drives you toward your goal. Willpower, on the other hand, is the "how". It's about self-control, discipline and the ability to manage distractions. Think of motivation as the engine of a car driving you towards your destination, whereas willpower is the steering wheel, helping you stay on course amidst a road filled with lots and swerves.

2.5. Understanding the Limits of Willpower

Like a battery, willpower drains, but it can also be recharged and strengthened. Repeatedly resisting temptation and focusing on tasks can consume your store of willpower, making self-control more difficult as the day wears on—a phenomenon referred to as 'ego depletion'. Understanding this 'limited resource model' of willpower has profound implications; it helps you strategize your day, prioritize tasks that need higher self-control, and time your breaks to recharge your willpower reserves.

2.6. The Science of Improving Willpower

Science also lends advice on amplifying one's willpower. Techniques vary from improving physical health, through regular exercise and a balanced diet, to adopting mindfulness practices, such as meditation, which train the brain for better self-control. Maintaining a stable sleep schedule is another proven strategy.

2.7. Transforming Life with the Power of Willpower

The power of willpower extends far beyond individual successes. When harnessed, it can lead to transformative changes in communities and societies, broadening its scope from personal growth to societal progress. Each goal achieved through determination and self-control, contributes to a grander vision, setting the stage for a chain reaction of positive transformations.

As the journey of demystifying willpower continues, it's crucial to recognize its transformative potential. Chapter two will delve much deeper into the biology behind willpower, providing further insights into how this potent tool is a result of not just our psychological but also biological processes. Understanding the power of willpower is the first step on this absorbing journey. Armed with this knowledge, you are now ready to forge ahead and learn more about exploiting this exceptional strength within you.

Chapter 3. The Biology of Willpower: A Deeper Look

In order to fully grasp the concept of willpower, we must first delve into its biological origins. Psychology and neuroscience have made incredible strides over the past few decades in uncovering the neural mechanisms and biological underpinnings of willpower. This exploration will marry these sciences and enable a vivid picture of how our bodies and brains enable us to make choices, resist temptations, and persist in the face of struggles.

3.1. The Brain and Willpower

Our brain is unequivocally the command center of the body. It harbors a multitude of interconnected regions, each with its own unique function, intricately working in sync to influence our thoughts, actions, emotions, and indeed, our willpower. Willpower, is associated largely with a part of the brain known as the prefrontal cortex, more specifically, its anterior cingulate cortex (ACC) and the dorsolateral prefrontal cortex (dlPFC) regions.

The prefrontal cortex—the forehead's front part—is responsible for our ability to think and plan, manage emotional responses, make decisions, and exhibit self-control or willpower. The ACC assists in monitoring conflicts, detecting errors, and assessing potential rewards or punishments, while the dlPFC plays a crucial role in maintaining focus and managing cognitive tasks, including directing willpower and mitigating impulsive behavior.

But what makes the prefrontal cortex tick? How does it regulate our willpower? The key lies in the rich cocktail of neurotransmitters, chemicals vital to transmitting information across the brain's structure and affecting our behavior.

3.2. Neurotransmitters: Agents of Willpower

Neurotransmitters are essentially the brain's chemical messengers. They facilitate communication between neurons by crossing the synapse — the tiny gap separating neurons. Among them, dopamine and serotonin are significant players in the willpower arena.

Dopamine, often coined the 'reward molecule', is deeply entwined with our motivation, pleasure, and reward system. It fuels our desires and encourages us to repeat actions that satiate those desires by activating a pleasant emotional response. Despite its rewarding benefits, dopamine can become a double-edged sword if not well controlled, pushing individuals towards addictive behaviors.

Serotonin, the 'feel-good neurotransmitter,' impacts mood, desire, and appetite. A balanced serotonin level generates feelings of happiness and well-being, regulates sleep and appetite, and influences our general mood. It's also known to inhibit impulsive behavior, hence playing a vital role in willpower.

3.3. The Neural Pathway of Willpower

The brain has a unique 'boost mode' for willpower. When faced with a challenge or temptation, our body initiates a fascinating domino effect. The prefrontal cortex gets activated, dopamine and serotonin levels adjust for optimal motivation and cognitive control, and a cascade of activities in the brain's neural networks reinforce our resolve, empowering an increase in willpower.

3.4. The Role of Glucose

Glucose—the body's main energy source—plays a significant role in willpower. Our brain, despite being only 2% of our body weight, consumes about 20% of our daily energy intake. Glucose fuels all brain activity, including the exertion of willpower. Studies suggest it might act as a kind of short-term reserve, which depletes upon activation of willpower. Forethought towards maintaining stable glucose levels could help maintain willpower strength throughout any given day.

3.5. Hormonal Influence

Hormones also play a crucial role in our willpower. The delicate dance of hormones like cortisol and insulin influences glucose regulation and stress response, both substantial willpower contributors. A balanced hormonal harmony can bolster resistance against impulsive decisions and reinforce our commitment to goals.

The journey in unlocking the biology of willpower is a fascinating one, granting us insights into our vibrant inner workings and how our bodies and minds symbiotically intertwine to influence our behavior. Remember, harnessing willpower is a lifetime endeavor. Stay patient with your progress; small, consistent steps often lead to significant leaps in personal growth. Armed with this knowledge, you are poised to better understand your willpower, and in tandem, navigate your path towards unshakeable commitment.

Chapter 4. Exploring Internal Motivations: The Fuel of Commitment

Motivation, the catalyst for every endeavor we undertake, the invisible hand that propels us forward, is a complex phenomenon intimately interwoven with the fabric of our consciousness. It's an element that lies at the foundation of our willpower, providing sustenance, strength, and vigor to our resolve, and enabling us to set our sights on a goal and strive relentlessly towards its fulfillment. When we endeavor to comprehend the significance of our motivations, we often find ourselves engulfed in a sea of questions, each leading further into the labyrinth of the human psyche. To unravel this enigma and better understand the intricacies of what drives us, a concept known as internal or intrinsic motivation comes into play.

4.1. Understanding Internal Motivation

Once we peel back the outer layer of motivation — the incentives and rewards that compel us to act — we uncover a deeper stratum: internal motivation. At its core, internal motivation is cut from the same cloth as self-determinism and autonomy. It originates within ourselves, not dependent on external factors or rewards. It's the impulse we feel when we engage in an activity for sheer joy, fulfillment, or because we deem it morally or ethically right. It's the music that a composer creates not for recognition or profit, but for the sheer thrill of bringing a melody to life, the fervent study of a biologist driven by an insatiable quest for knowledge, or the voluntary contributions of a philanthropist committed to alleviating societal hardships.

Internal motivations are powered by three fundamental elements: autonomy, competence, and relatedness. Autonomy, the desire for self-governance, gives us the freedom to choose our paths. Competence, the need to master our sphere, brings fulfillment through growth and self-improvement. Relatedness, the longing for meaningful relationships and connections, enhances our sense of belongingness.

4.2. Fanning the Flames of Intrinsic Drive

Harnessing internal motivation is akin to tending to a fire within our psyche. It must be kindled carefully, fueled diligently, and its flames fanned regularly. Otherwise, it may falter. Here are some strategies to stoke the embers of your intrinsic drive.

Self-Exploration: Delve deeper into your mind to discover what sparks joy, interest, or curiosity in you. Your internal motivations are closely tied to your deepest passions and inclinations. Identifying and aligning yourself with these internal drives can lay the foundation for a willpower characterized by unswerving commitment.

Goal Setting: Once you've identified your internal motivations, translate them into actionable goals. Ensure these objectives are Specifically-defined, Measurable, Achievable, Relevant, and Time-bound (SMART). Such an approach ensures clarity, facilitating focus and driving forward motion.

Celebrate Progress: Celebrating your victories, however small, fuels self-satisfaction, revitalizing your internal motivation. Develop a system to track and celebrate your progress towards your goals. This could be as simple as maintaining a journal or using a digital tool.

4.3. The Power of Intrinsic Motivation in Fostering Willpower

Deep-seated internal motivation sets the stage for powerful willpower. It uniquely fortifies your resilience, equipping you to overcome challenges, manage setbacks, and persist in your pursuit. Since it is internally-authored, it's more sustainable, not susceptible to external influences such as fluctuating rewards or recognition.

People with high internal motivation are typically self-initiators, able to sustain action even in the absence of immediate rewards. As such, internal motivation serves as a nourishing reservoir from which our willpower can continually draw strength, fueling our commitment and enhancing the likelihood of success.

4.4. Case Study: Examining Internal Motivation in Action

Consider the story of Mary, a corporate executive who harbored a deeply-felt inclination towards learning. Rather than seeking promotions or raises, what fascinated her most was the acquisition and application of knowledge. This internal motivation saw her relentlessly devour books, attend seminars and engage in online courses. Over time, her wealth of knowledge proved invaluable, earning her the respect of her colleagues and superiors. Proving her ability to learn complex topics proficiently, she was presented with challenging projects and leadership responsibilities, eventually find herself at the helm of the company. Mary's story is testament to the power of internal motivation; it was her fuel of commitment that stoked the flames of her willpower, driving her to persevere and ultimately succeed.

4.5. Conclusion: Unleashing the Force of Your Inner Drive

As we culminate this exploration into the realm of internal motivations and their profound impact on shaping willpower, it becomes evident how closely our commitment and resilience are tied to our innermost desires and passions. By identifying these underlying drivers, nurturing them, and channelizing them towards unfolding our potential, we can wield our willpower like never before, turning the art of unbreakable commitment from an elusive ideal to a tangible reality.

In the end, the journey to empowered willpower is rooted deeply within us, within our motivation and our commitment to pursuing this internal motivation. It is an inward journey — a journey that requires introspection, identification of our deepest desires, and their careful nurturing. It's far from easy, but its rewards are precious. For, in unlocking our internal motivations, we do not just develop an iron will; we devise a powerful engine that can drive us unfailingly towards our dreams and aspirations.

Chapter 5. Cultivating Unbreakable Commitment: Strategies and Techniques

Undoubtedly, commitment is a powerful tool, a dynamic force propelling you towards realizing your dreams and objectives. But, what happens when commitment wanes? How do we cultivate unbreakable commitment that stands firm regardless of the trials and tribulations thrown our way? This chapter details a series of potent strategies and techniques designed to fortify your commitment, ensuring that it doesn't just endure, but flourishes under any circumstances.

5.1. Identifying Core Values

One of the elemental foundation stones for building unbreakable commitment lies in recognizing your core values. These are fundamental beliefs and principles that guide your actions and decisions. They are the why behind what we do, acting as our internal compass guiding us in life. To identify these, question what is truly important to you. What principles do you live by? What makes you feel emotionally fulfilled? Take time to introspect and note down these values. Reflect on them and understand how they shape your life and actions.

5.2. Uncovering Your Why

Your reasoning, or 'why', fuels commitment. This 'why' is your deep-seated motivator that keeps you pressing forward, even in the face of adversity. Explore what is truly motivating you to reach your goals. Is it personal achievement? Recognition? Financial stability? Anchor your commitment to this reason and remind yourself of it daily. It will serve as the underpinning of your unyielding determination.

5.3. Setting Clear, Realistic Goals

Setting clear and realistic goals gives you a sense of direction. Setting unattainable goals can lead to failure and disrupt your commitment. Thus, it's critical to set goals that motivate you and are realistically attainable. Use the SMART technique: Specific, Measurable, Achievable, Relevant, and Time-bound goals. It provides an efficient framework to formulate your objectives, driving your commitment towards success.

5.4. Implementing Emotional Management

Commitment can be impacted by your emotional state. There will be days filled with positivity, and others clouded with negativity. Emotional management helps steady your emotions and reinforce your commitment during difficult times. Practice mindfulness, gratitude, and resilience to ensure your emotions align with your commitment rather than act against it. Remember, emotions can either fuel or deplete your commitment; it's down to your ability to manage them effectively.

5.5. Creating a Supportive Environment

Our surroundings hugely influence our commitment. If you're immersed in a supportive environment that promotes our values and goals, it's easier to stay committed. Surround yourself with people who encourage and inspire you, leverage tools and resources that facilitate your commitment, and disassociate from distractions that could potentially erode your determination.

5.6. Adopting a Growth Mindset

Develop a growth mindset, where challenges are seen as opportunities for improvement rather than insurmountable obstacles. This perspective hinges on the belief that our capabilities and skills can be developed over time through hard work, practice, and consistent learning. Embrace the journey with all its ups and downs, certain in the knowledge that each trial is making you stronger, and your commitment unbreakable.

5.7. Continuous Learning and Improvement

Value learning and constant improvement. Knowledge is power, providing you with the tools and techniques to navigate your path to success. Embrace new skills, take risks, and learn from your failures. Make it a habit to learn something new each day, no matter how small; this will fuel your curiosity, keep you engaged and as a result, fortify your commitment.

5.8. Embrace Failure as a Stepping Stone

One of the most challenging things in life is facing failure. However, it's an indispensable stage of growth. Look at it as a learning opportunity rather than an end. Be tenacious. Understand and analyze your failures; they offer valuable insights and lessons that will allow you to adapt, evolve and heighten your path to success.

In conclusion, to foster unshakeable commitment, you need to understand your core values, find your 'why', set clear, realistic goals, manage your emotions, create a conducive environment, have a growth mindset, constantly learn, improve, and view failure as a stepping stone. Incorporate these strategies and techniques into your daily life, and witness a significant boost in your resolve, taking you one step closer to achieving your dreams. As Aristotle says 'we are what we repeatedly do. Excellence, therefore, is not an act but a habit.' Here's to crafting the habit of unbreakable commitment!

Chapter 6. Harnessing Self-Discipline: Building Blocks of Willpower

Adorning the cape of self-discipline is pivotal in forging a robust willpower. It requires dedicated commitment, but it fortifies your mindset, nourishing the seed of determination into a robust tree of steadfastness. In this discourse, we delve into several techniques and strategies that guide you towards embracing the virtue of self-discipline. Strategic themes are structured into the exploration of 'What,' 'Why,' and 'How' attached to self-discipline, its benefits, and harnessing its potent influence on willpower respectively.

6.1. What is Self-Discipline?

Self-discipline, often analogous to self-control, is the ability to align one's day-to-day decisions with their overall long-term goals. It manifests as the restraint demonstrated towards one's impulses and relies less on immediate gratification for longer-term benefits. Self-discipline is a muscle: the more you flex it, the stronger it becomes. Its cultivation transforms mundane routine into a disciplined regimen and impacts choices, thereby working towards the grander picture of self-improvement.

6.2. Importance of Self-Discipline

Recognizing the critical role of self-discipline expedites the journey towards achieving unyielding willpower. Self-discipline is a potent antidote to procrastination that weakens resolve. It fosters time management, improves decision-making ability, and promotes mental stability. It fuels the journey towards self-actualization and accomplishment, paving the path for superior goal orientation. When paired with a clear vision, it transforms intangible aspirations into tangible experiences.

6.3. Strategies to Develop Self-Discipline

The core of our exploration settles on practical strategies and techniques to nurture self-discipline effectively. The approach to building self-discipline varies significantly from person to person; however, there are universally applicable steps designed to steer you in the right direction:

1. Identification of Weaknesses: The first stride towards development always involves self-awareness. Recognize and understand your weaknesses that succumb to instant gratification. Only then can you effectively devise strategies to overcome them.

2. Setting Clear Goals: Utilize, 'SMART' (Specific, Measurable, Achievable, Relevant, and Time-bound) goals to scrutinize both long-term and short-term aspirations. This keeps you focused and facilitates constructive progress.

3. Progress Tracking: Regular check-ins on your progress reinforces motivation, and highlights the areas requiring additional attention. This could be maintained in the form of a simple diary or a more detailed planner.

4. Building Routines: Consistency is the bedrock of self-discipline. By establishing a routine, discipline is exercised daily. This could be as simple as a morning workout or dedicating specific time for reading.

5. Cultivating Patience: Results do not surface immediately and expecting them to lead to heightened dissatisfaction. Understand that self-discipline is a gradual process and appreciate the small successes along your journey.

6.4. Impact of Self-Discipline on Willpower

Self-discipline fortifies willpower and helps in maintaining a steady resolve. With improved self-discipline, you are better at withstanding temptations and are less likely to indulge in actions that diminish your mental energy. Strong self-discipline consequently begets enhanced willpower, favoring both personal growth and professional development.

6.5. The Mechanics of Discipline and Willpower

The relationship between discipline and willpower is intrinsically intertwining. Disciplined individuals don't rely solely on willpower to guide their decisions. Instead, self-discipline enhances the practical application of willpower. Disciplined behaviors become automatic over time, reducing the need to exercise willpower. This mechanism not only conserves mental energy but also fortifies the reserves of willpower for times when it's needed most.

6.6. Using Willpower Wisely

For all its worth, willpower is not an infinite resource. Conscious attention towards its targeted application pays dividends in the long run. Understand that all tasks do not require equal applications of willpower. Prioritize and allocate your willpower reserves accordingly. Similarly, the relation between willpower and physical health is reciprocal. Adequate rest, regular exercise, and a balanced diet replenish willpower reserves, while also enhancing the ability to exert self-control.

This carefully crafted exploration acts as a profound guide for harnessing self-discipline, the quintessential building block of willpower. Embrace these strategies to foster a stalwart commitment in your pursuit of excellence. By understanding, prioritizing, and cultivating discipline, you augment your reservoir of willpower, propelling you towards actualizing your full potential. It's about valuing the journey over the destination, and valuing the willpower built along the way.

Chapter 7. Overcoming Procrastination: Tactics for Success

Among all the roadblocks to the development of willpower and steadfast commitment, procrastination stands as a formidable foe. In this chapter, we delve into this prevalent issue, demystifying its origins and patterns, and arming you with effective strategies and tips to minimize its impact on your productivity and drive.

7.1. Unearthing the Roots of Procrastination

Procrastination, in its simplest form, is the act of delaying tasks or actions. But beneath the surface of this seemingly benign behavior lie more complex psychological and emotional factors. Studies suggest that procrastination might be due, in part, to brain chemistry, particularly activities in the limbic system (the pleasure center) and the prefrontal cortex (the decision-making center). Essentially, when the desire for immediate pleasure overpowers the logic of future benefits, procrastination sets in. But fear not, it's possible to rewire these adverse patterns and cultivate a mindset conducive to goal-oriented action.

7.2. Strategies to Overcome Procrastination

To overcome procrastination, you need systematic and consistent efforts. Here are a few practical strategies designed to combat this insidious habit and empower you towards achieving your goals:

Break Down Goals into Manageable Tasks: Large or complex tasks can trigger overwhelm, leading to procrastination. Breaking down your overarching goals into smaller, manageable tasks makes them appear less intimidating, encouraging you to start working on them.

Prioritize Tasks: Determine the urgency and importance of each task, ranking them in a priority list. Attend to high-priority tasks first and avoid wasting time on less critical tasks until the important ones are completed.

Set Clear Deadlines: Deadlines create a sense of urgency and compel you to act. Be specific about when you'll complete each task, but maintain flexibility to adapt to changes and unforeseen work.

Establish a Routine: Establish a dedicated work routine and stick to it. Consistency mitigates the emotional discomfort associated with tackling difficult tasks.

7.3. The Power of Time Management

Effective time management significantly reduces procrastination. It enables you to organise your tasks in a structured manner, minimising the likelihood of you prioritising non-essential tasks over tasks pertinent to your goals. Consider these tools for effective time management:

Time-Blocking: Allocate specific time slots to tasks. Time-blocking promotes focus by creating psychological commitment to a task during its appointed slot.

Pomodoro Technique: This method involves breaking your work into intervals of concentrated work, typically 25 minutes, followed by a short break. It's an effective way to manage mental energy and reduce fatigue.

Eisenhower Box: This tool helps you decide on and prioritize tasks by urgency and importance, sorting out less urgent and important tasks which you should either delegate or not do at all.

7.4. Leveraging Technology to Combat Procrastination

Today's technological advancements offer multiple ways to assist in overcoming procrastination. Apps and software designed to increase productivity can be a game-changer for individuals battling procrastination. Some popular options include:

Task Management Tools: Apps like Trello, Asana, or Todoist help organize tasks in an easy-to-view format.

Time Trackers: Tools like RescueTime, Clockify, or Toggl Track offer comprehensive insights into your daily routines and work habits.

Focus Apps: Apps such as Forest and Focus@Will can aid in maintaining focus by minimizing distractions.

7.5. Addressing Emotional Factors

Recognize that emotional factors often underlie procrastination. Emotions such as fear of failure, self-doubt, and perfectionism can sabotage your progress and need to be addressed. Practices like mindfulness meditation, regular exercises, and employing a growth mindset can alleviate these emotional roadblocks.

7.6. Creating an Environment Conducive to Action

Your environment influences your behaviour to a great extent. A well-organized, distraction-free workspace can enhance focus and reduce the likelihood of procrastination.

By addressing procrastination and implementing these tactics for success, you are taking a significant step towards improving your willpower and commitment. Remember, patience and consistency are key to this journey. Don't be discouraged by setbacks. Instead, view them as opportunities to learn and grow. With time and dedicated effort, you will harness the power to overcome procrastination, and move steadfastly towards your goals.

Chapter 8. The Role of Habits in Fostering Strong Willpower

Mastering the labyrinthine channels of willpower unquestionably requires a deep comprehension of an integral aspect of our daily lives: our habits. Just as the steady flow of a river inevitably etches a path into the landscape, the rhythmic cadence of our habits carves significant imprints into the terrain of our minds. These recurrent patterns of thought and behavior are powerful forces: they have the capacity to undermine our resolve, but they can just as easily be bent towards fostering robust willpower when properly understood and harnessed.

8.1. The Mechanics Of Habits

Habits are not random phenomena; they are derived from distinct processes within our brains. A habit is composed of three elements: the cue, the routine, and the reward. The cue is a trigger that initiates the habit, the routine is the action taken, and the reward fulfills a desire, cementing the habit further in our minds. Despite them being deeply ingrained in our psyche, habits are susceptible to change by restructuring these component elements, a task made crucial in bolstering willpower.

8.2. The Double-Edged Sword of Habit

As omnipresent shapers of our daily lives, habits can take on two fundamentally oppositional roles. On one hand, they can act as obstinate barriers obstructing our path towards our desired future.

Whether it's a dependence on sweets when stressed, or the itch to check social media while studying, certain habits can hinder us from fully engaging our willpower.

On the other hand, habits also hold the potential to serve as powerful tools in magnifying our willpower. Designed thoughtfully, they can propel us towards our goals with a push akin to the wind filling the sails of a ship. These are productive habits, instilled deliberately with our objectives in mind.

8.3. Building Productive Habits

Productive habits are neither acquired overnight nor are they the result of fortuitous circumstances. Crafting these habits necessitates purposeful design, coupled with consistency in practice and the cognizance of patience.

In the context of building willpower, productive habits can range from daily meditation to strengthen mental fortitude, to planning your day the night before to better manage time, to regular exercise for increased mental stamina. The formation of such habits begins firstly by identifying productive routines that align with your goals, and then deliberately implanting cues and rewards to trigger and reinforce these routines.

8.4. Modifying Destructive Habits

Conquering willpower challenges frequently demands that we confront destructive habits head-on, and, when confrontation proves insufficient, to alter or replace these unproductive routines. To do so, we must delve into the anatomy of the habit, isolating the cues and rewards surrounding the detrimental routines.

Once we've identified the incentives and triggers of the habit, we can consciously replace the negative routine with a positive one, ensuring the substitute still meets the reward requirement. If, for instance, you notice you reach for your phone in response to boredom (the cue), try substituting scrolling through social media (destructive routine) with reading a few pages of an enlightening book (productive routine), promising similar gratification (reward).

8.5. Cultivating Habitual Awareness

A major step towards mastering habits lies in cultivating habitual awareness; that is, regularly examining your habits to evaluate their impact on your willpower. By understanding which habits prove empowering or disempowering, you can stay one step ahead in the battle between fleeting urges and long-term commitment. Maintain an observant eye on your routine to grasp how, and which, habits significantly affect your willpower.

8.6. Habits: The Bridge to Strong Willpower

In essence, considering the integral role habits play, they can be envisioned as architects of our future selves. By consciously curating a pattern of productive habits, while modifying or eliminating the destructive ones, we lay the foundation for an unassailable fortress of willpower. An intentional and disciplined relationship with our habits can indeed turn our pursuits of resilience and fortitude from a struggle into a storyline of personal transformation and victories. A self-aware, dedicated approach towards our habitual patterns can illuminate the path to a more disciplined, committed, and willful life.

In closing, it may be said that our habits are the notes to the symphony of our willpower. Played discordantly, they can create cacophonous noise, jarring our resolve off its track. But when harmonized with precision, they form a melodious tune that propels us fluidly through the pages of our personal journey.

The power to fabricate strong willpower lies not only in understanding how to resist temptations and overcome uncertainties but also in learning how to navigate the subtle undercurrents of our habits. Thus, to foster strong willpower, we have to amend our 'scripts' of habits and retune them to our advantage. Remember, this is not a simple or quick process, but a journey that requires persistence, patience, and, above all, a firm commitment to continual growth and transformation.

Taken together, the heartening message is clear: With wilful persistence, you have the power to turn the gears of habits to your will. Today's struggle is the architect of an empowered 'you' of tomorrow. The lessons you've learned in this journey are signposts, marking the trail toward the pinnacle of self-mastery and unyielding determination. As you stride forward, remember: A change in habit heralds a change in life. Let this understanding serve as a beacon, guiding your steps toward a steadfast commitment – the unbreakable signature of extraordinary willpower.

Chapter 9. Resilience and Persistence: The Art of Bouncing Back

Resilience and persistence are the two indispensable facets of an unshakable willpower that serve as the foundation for any long-lasting commitment. As we explore these foundational elements, remember that your journey towards an unbreakable commitment is unique to you. Personal growth requires no fixed route; you chart the course.

9.1. " The Twin Pillars of Resilience and Persistence"

Resilience is the art of bouncing back from adversity, trials, and setbacks. It is the ability to continue moving forward with unwavering focus while maintaining a positive attitude. On the other hand, persistence is a steadfast quality that keeps you going against all odds, convincing you to never give up despite the magnitude of the challenges you face. Together, resilience and persistence create an unbreakable tag-team of positive mindset and relentless forward motion – the potent combination needed to forge ahead, especially when enduring the tough path to your envisioned future.

Initially, it is important to establish that setbacks are a natural part of life. They do not stand to define us, yet how we respond to these adversities does. The amalgamation of resilience and persistence assists in creating a healthy and robust response to life's inevitable hurdles.

9.2. " Understanding the Dance Between Resilience and Persistence"

The synergy between resilience and persistence can be described as an intricate dance. While resilience absorbs the impact of the setbacks, enabling an individual to maintain a positive mental state and recover quickly, persistence assures that the person continues their journey, focusing on the goal tirelessly. This undeterred focus enables continued action towards the purpose, without being derailed by adversity, which is the essence of real progress.

Resilience, in essence, promotes psychologically healthy mechanisms to cope with, recover from, and thrive in the face of adversity. Meanwhile, persistence can be likened to an internal engine that keeps your actions aligned with your purpose, regardless of the number of roadblocks encountered. The close-knit relationship between these two defining characteristics is therefore instrumental in overcoming adversities and upholding commitments.

9.3. " Cultivating Resilience: Embracing the Ebb and Flow"

Resilience is a powerful emotional resource that can be nurtured and cultivated. It is born out of a mindset that views challenges not as overwhelming threats, but as opportunities for growth and character-building. To enhance your resilience, work on developing a positive and adaptive attitude towards life's adversities.

A primary step is to embrace the reality that life fluctuates between highs and lows, recognizing that setbacks and difficulties are not aberrations, but integral to the human experience. This acceptance encourages us to develop resilience as a tool for navigating life's inevitable storms.

To further develop your resilience, commit to nurturing your emotional well-being. Prioritize self-care, engage in activities that promote self-compassion, and develop your emotional intelligence. Furthermore, develop relationships that are meaningful and supportive, as they create a safety net that can prove indispensable in your journey towards magnified resilience.

9.4. " Fueling Persistence: Keeping Your Eyes on the Prize"

While resilience is about swift recovery from adversity, persistence is your unwavering dedication to the achievement of a worthwhile goal. It is crucial to remember that the journey's length or the roadblocks it contains do not influence the worthiness of your purpose.

To boost your persistence, firstly, clearly laid down goals are essential. With cogent goals outlined, your persistence finds a direction, propelling you forwards. Secondly, develop optimism, as maintaining an optimistic perspective even in daunting situations fuels the persistence needed to carry on. Be persistent in your optimism too, persistently finding reasons to stay hopeful.

Additionally, maintain flexible strategies. Rather than viewing shifts in strategy as a setback, view them as necessary adaptations for progress. This strategy promotes persistence, as it reframes setbacks into opportunities to learn and grow.

In conclusion, resilience and persistence are two sides of a powerful coin that fuels an unshakeably dedicated commitment. It is a dance between bouncing back and moving forwards, continuously adapting and growing. Through the cultivation of both resilience and persistence, you foster an inherent ability to sustain your focus and alignment towards your goals, enhancing your journey to personal growth and indomitable perseverance. Following these guidance, you can thrive in the face of adversity, transform setbacks into comebacks, and place one foot in front of the other persistently, nurturing an unbreakable commitment to your future.

Chapter 10. Case Studies: Triumph of Willpower and Commitment

In the evocative landscape of willpower and commitment, there are stories abound that serve as shining beacons of inspiration and profound learning. Hand-picked from a ceaseless ocean of human threshold, the case studies presented here act as mirrors, reflecting evolved definitions of resolve, focus, grit, and ambition. Torsos hardened by the unyielding steel of willpower, these narratives are more than just bedtime stories—they are transformative life lessons that have the power to help you reshape your own destiny.

10.1. The Everest Triumph: Sir Edmund Hillary and Tenzing Norgay

Ascending the height of a whopping 8,848 meters, this first tale begins on the frosty summit of Mount Everest. Sir Edmund Hillary, a zealous mountaineer from New Zealand, and Tenzing Norgay, a steadfast Sherpa from Nepal, etched a new chapter in the books of human achievement on May 29, 1953, when they successfully summited the Earth's highest peak.

Their expedition was not just a test of physical endurance but an exemplar of relentless willpower. Undeterred by past failures, they confronted bone-chilling winds, menacing crevasses, avalanche-prone routes, and dwindling oxygen levels. Their unbreakable commitment was the essential cornerstone that led to their monumental success. This expedition underlines the pivotal role of unyielding willpower that can spur individuals to conquer towering challenges and etch their names in the annals of history.

10.2. The 4-Minute Mile: Sir Roger Bannister

Next, we set our focus on the lush green track where Sir Roger Bannister, an aspiring British athlete, quashed the longstanding myth that the human body was incapable of running a mile in less than 4 minutes. On May 6, 1954, Bannister accomplished this seemingly impossible feat, clocking in at 3 minutes and 59.4 seconds.

Average onlookers labeled this task as impossible. Bannister, however, was far from disheartened. His audacious belief in his abilities and an unbreakable commitment to his ambition fueled his willpower. His relentless training coupled with his unwavering will led him to shatter the 4-minute barrier. Bannister's tale serves as a compelling reminder that willpower, combined with a determined mindset, can help us transcend the boundaries of presumed human limitations.

10.3. J.K Rowling's Spellbinding Persistence

Now, let's traverse the world of literature. J.K. Rowling, the renowned author of the Harry Potter series, endured numerous rejections before she tasted success. At one point, her life was mired in single motherhood, divorce, and near-poverty.

The seemingly insoluble challenges did not deter her. On the contrary, they fueled her willpower, and she took to writing with an unshakable commitment. Seven years after she started writing, she eventually received her first acceptance from Bloomsbury Publishing House. Rowling's journey highlights that perseverance in the face of adversity, driven by indomitable willpower, can carve the path to phenomenal success.

10.4. Reinvention of Steve Jobs

The final stop of our case study journey lies in the heart of Silicon Valley. Steve Jobs, the mastermind behind Apple Inc., faced a humiliating ouster from his own company in 1985. This event could have spelled the end of an extraordinary career for many, but not Jobs.

Strengthened by willpower and an unbreakable resolve, Jobs founded NeXT Inc., an innovative but underappreciated computer platform. This experience was pivotal, marking a transformative phase in Jobs's career. When Apple found itself on the brink of bankruptcy, Jobs was called back to steer the sinking ship, and he orchestrated an astonishing turnaround for the company. His extraordinary journey delineates how people with unsuspected reserves of willpower, bolstered by an unshakable commitment, can alter their destiny and impact the world.

In conclusion, these case studies are vivid illustrations of the triumph of willpower and commitment. Each story gives us valuable insights into how unwavering resolve, coupled with indomitable willpower, can help us surmount obstacles, achieve our goals and reshape our future. These narratives encourage us to tap into our reservoir of willpower, catalyze an unshakable commitment to our aspirations, thus leading us down the path of personal and professional growth. Through these case studies, we learn to triumph over our circumstances, transform everyday struggles into opportunities, and march forward undaunted, with an iron will and an unflinching spirit.

Chapter 11. Roadmap to a Powerful Future: Maintaining Your Unbreakable Commitment

The concluding chapter of our special report, "Roadmap to a Powerful Future: Maintaining Your Unbreakable Commitment," ushers a comprehensive exploration into the dynamics of sustaining your willpower and dedication over the long haul. We are leaving the realm of abstract theories and entering the world of tangible plans—plans that will guide you toward a future brimming with power and commitment.

11.1. Establishing Your Willpower Manifesto

As you venture into solidifying your strong willpower, an essential first step is drafting a clear, cogent "Willpower Manifesto." This document encapsulates the principles that guide your journey. In writing this, consider your values, strengths, and aspirations. Reflect on your journey thus far, the challenges you've overcome, and those you might encounter. The Willpower Manifesto should rekindle your commitment every time you read it. It isn't etched in stone but evolves as you grow and learn, open to refinements that echo your unfolding understanding.

11.2. The Power of Regular Reflection

Strategically pause and assess your progress at regular intervals. This habitual introspection can help identify potential pitfalls, celebrate achievements, and renew your commitment. One of the most effective ways to incorporate reflection is through journaling. Journaling enables you to document your journey, chronicle successes, and express frustrations, all while helping you cultivate a clear, articulate voice of inner dialogue.

11.3. Courage in the Face of Setbacks

Every path to success is laden with obstacles and setbacks. Instead of allowing these incidents to demotivate you, use them as stepping stones towards your unshakeable commitment. Understand that failure is not a sign of weakness, but evidence of strength and perseverance. Cultivate resilience, bounce back with even more determination, and continue to move forward, undeterred by the hurdles of life.

11.4. Continuous Learning: A Key to Maintaining Commitment

Never stop learning. New knowledge and experiences can dramatically reinvigorate your sense of purpose and stoke the fires of your commitment. For instance, you might find new research on willpower or discover an inspiring story about the triumph of tenacity over adversity. These new insights and perspectives can provide fresh ammunition for your arsenal of willpower and commitment.

11.5. Cultivating A Supportive Environment

Surround yourself with individuals who support and inspire you. Create an environment that fosters growth and fuels your commitment. Should you encounter setbacks, these individuals can provide motivation, practical advice, and emotional support. They can reinvigorate your energy, inspire you, and help you maintain your unbreakable commitment.

11.6. Ensuring Work-Life Balance

Maintaining your willpower does not mean completely sidelining leisure or neglecting other life aspects. Striking a healthy work-life balance ensures that your willpower doesn't lead to burnout. This balance allows you to give adequate attention to personal relationships, hobbies, and relaxation while upholding your commitment.

11.7. The Power of Reward: Celebrate Small Wins

Recognizing and celebrating small achievements is crucial to maintaining momentum. Whether it's reaching a minor milestone or conquering a challenging situation, acknowledging your victories stokes self-esteem and motivates continued adherence to your commitment.

11.8. A Lifetime Journey

Maintaining an unbreakable commitment is not a task you complete and check off; it's a life-long journey. Traditional "end point" thinking can lead to a sense of disappointment if progress is slow. Instead, cultivate the mindset that you are on an unending journey, continuously evolving, learning, and improving. Your willpower and commitment should be flexible, adjusting to align with your journey's dynamic nature.

Remember, the journey to unshakeable commitment demands time, patience, and dedication. This roadmap will guide you, empowering you to forge an unwavering commitment to achieve your heartfelt aspirations. Sturdy willpower, resilient commitment, and a frame of mind tempered by experience – these tools form the cornerstone of your powerful future. Embrace this journey wholeheartedly and let the voyages into the depths of your willpower begin!